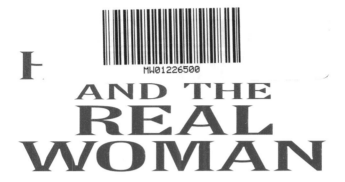

6.25

H

AND THE
REAL
WOMAN

The Christian Science Publishing Society
Boston, Massachusetts, U.S.A.

INTRODUCTION

What is a *real* woman, and where does she find health and happiness in today's fast-paced world? The answers come in knowing what genuine well-being actually is and in understanding that *where* we look matters.

As one of the writers in this pamphlet writes, "The qualities of true womanhood — and manhood — are really inherent in all of us, because our genuine selfhood is the reflection of our Father-Mother God. Understanding and claiming this spiritual fact can enlarge the horizon of our thinking with a powerfully freeing effect on our lives."

OTHER
PUBLICATIONS
OF INTEREST

- A Letter to Someone in Love
- Beyond age, beyond time*
- Christian Science class instruction: Nurturing the desire to heal
- Church: A moral and spiritual force in the community
- God's Law of Adjustment/Possession*
- Home: "The dearest spot on earth"
- Human rights—a higher view
- Jobs, Careers, and Our Father's Business*
- Peace in the Neighborhood*
- Safety Assured*

*Available as pamphlet or cassette

CONTENTS

Articles adapted for publication in pamphlet format.

Health, happiness, and the body

One wonders whether all the information saturating our society — especially information about the body — can really significantly improve the quality of our lives. So much of the world's thinking today is centered on the body — its health, its beauty, its weight, its physical condition, what we should eat, and what we shouldn't eat.

An article in *Forbes* magazine concludes, "We are thinking thin and getting fat."[1] The article brings out that despite the relentless urging of health professionals and despite all the advertising that would push people to be more lean and fit, Americans are, on the whole, not finding the task easy.

And there's so much about exercise. We shouldn't get too little exercise — or too much. And then there's the verdict that certain kinds of exercise could be dangerous. Perhaps the lesson in all this is that the real answers to questions about fitness are not to be found where we're being instructed to look for them — in the body.

Most people think of the body as self-acting and also as subject to unseen and unknown forces that can invade it. Either way, it's believed that we can be victimized by our bodies. Everywhere we turn, we're confronted with the belief that the body is the source of our health and our happiness. But there's a different way of looking at our identity. In spite of all the enormous amounts of human information at our disposal and all the ready avenues for receiving it, the best — the basic — place to look for information vital to our well-being is still the inspired Word of the Bible. For example, the Bible tells us that man is the image and likeness of God and has dominion over all God's creation.[2]

Is that how we perceive ourselves — as wholly Godlike, entirely spiritual? Or do we think of ourselves as merely physical or perhaps as part physical, part mental?

Mary Baker Eddy, the Discoverer and Founder of Christian Science, writes in *Science and Health with Key to the Scriptures,* "The description of man as purely physical, or as both material and spiritual, — but in either case dependent upon his physical organization, — is the Pandora box, from which all ills have gone forth, especially despair."[3] The view of man as dependent on the body does bring despair. But the view of man put forth in the first chapter of the Bible includes dominion. So we have a choice: despair or dominion.

Is the body really our identity? In the Bible St. Paul encourages us to be "willing rather to be absent from the body, and to be present with the Lord."[4]

Imagine what could happen if we were to spend time each day with thought centered not on ourselves but on God — not passively but actively — hours spent not thinking of ourselves but learning more of God and actively expressing the qualities we associate with God: genuine love, patience, forgiveness, justice, joy.

Mrs. Eddy writes, "To live so as to keep human consciousness in constant relation with the divine, the spiritual, and the eternal, is to individualize infinite power; and this is Christian Science."[5] Thought centered on God instead of self doesn't neglect the body.

In fact, it helps care for — restore and heal — it. Through this spiritual view the body actually improves.

In the Bible we read, "To be carnally minded is death; but to be spiritually minded is life and peace."[6] To be spiritually-minded means to view things on the basis of spiritual reality instead of on the basis of appearance. Christ Jesus admonished, "Judge not according to the appearance, but judge righteous judgement."[7] To be spiritually-minded is to see God — eternal Life, all-encompassing Love, the one all-inclusive, harmonious Being — as reality. And it means recognizing discord, pettiness, illness — whatever is unlike the divine nature — as provably without power. In the spiritually-minded consciousness, which is uplifted and at peace, the healing Christ — the power of God — is felt, and we can see who we really are.

Just as we can't depend on the body for health, so depending on it for happiness is unwise, too. Mrs. Eddy writes, "A false sense of what constitutes happiness is more disastrous to human progress than all that an enemy or enmity can obtrude upon the mind or engraft upon its purposes and achievements wherewith to obstruct life's joys and enhance its sorrows."[8] False concepts of where we gain our happiness are responsible for such things as pornography and drug addiction.

Then, how do we achieve genuine happiness? Through the spiritual, God-created view of man. Happiness can't actually change — can't come and go — because spiritual reality never changes. And that's because God, divine Principle, divine Love, never changes. Prayer — our endeavor to bring thought into conformity with this divine Principle — helps us to hold on to our joy even in the midst of challenges. In fact, joy is precisely what so often ends up pulling us out of a difficulty!

This is not a matter of just trying to tough things out. It is a matter of feeling genuine joy — true joy — because of our understanding of spiritual reality, which is always present.

A few years ago I became aware that I had a lump on my body. As a Christian Scientist I prayed to gain a clearer sense of spiritual reality. Later the condition started to be painful. So I got very still and listened. I had to admit that I was afraid. And then I realized that I was afraid I was going to die. But on the heels of that fear I suddenly thought, "All space is filled with God's love. There just isn't any way that I can possibly get outside of God's love. There is no way that I can ever be separated from God's love."

I had the most wonderful sense of being enveloped in God's love. It was a moment of pure joy and freedom. The fear and the anxiety left completely, and the pain was gone, too. I don't know when the lump disappeared, but it was soon gone. During those moments, I was so conscious of the infinitude of God's love — the all-encompassing love of God that enfolds the universe and from which we can never be separated — that there just wasn't any room for belief in pain or fear or disease symptoms.

Science and Health explains what happens at such times: "Become conscious for a single moment that Life and intelligence are purely spiritual, — neither in nor of matter — and the body will then utter no complaints. If suffering from a belief in sickness, you will find yourself suddenly well. Sorrow is turned into joy when the body is controlled by spiritual Life, Truth, and Love."[9]

We don't ever have to despair. Our bodies are not in control. God is in control. We're not dependent on our bodies for health or happiness. Our joy is already full because of who we really are: the spiritual image and likeness of God — pure, eternal, beautiful, expressing His goodness.

You know, that's the best information anyone could ever get.

[1]James Ring Adams and Jeffrey A. Trachtenberg, "Losing the battle of the bulge," *Forbes,* November 17, 1986, p. 172. [2]See Gen. 1:26. [3]*Science and Health,* p. 170. [4]II Cor. 5:8. [5]*The First Church of Christ, Scientist, and Miscellany,* p. 160. [6]Rom. 8:6. [7]John 7:24. [8]*Miscellaneous Writings,* pp. 9–10. [9]*Science and Health,* p. 14.

God causes health, not illness

One of the spiritual truths basing all Christian Science healing is this: God alone is the cause of all existence, and if God does not cause something, man cannot really experience it. God, good, is the creative Principle of all that actually exists. In the first chapter of Genesis we read of God creating man in His own image and likeness and making His entire creation good.[1]

When confronted by disease, one might begin by asking himself, Is God the cause of this? If God is good, He cannot cause evil, for this would mean that His power perpetuates evil instead of destroying it.

Next one might ask, Then is this sickness actually going on? Herein lies the crux of the whole problem. Physical sense testimony argues for the reality of the situation: the patient (oneself or another) is distressed, perhaps feverish and afraid. How can one say disease isn't going on? It looks and feels completely real. But on the basis that Principle, God, is good and the only cause, it cannot be true, and the seem-so should be surrendered to omnipotent Principle.

Yielding up any belief in disease as real and in suffering as a necessity, accepting the sublime fact that God, the only cause, is in control of His perfect effect, man, we have had "faith as a grain of mustard seed." This is the requirement for utilizing divine power, Christ Jesus assured us. "If ye have faith as a grain of mustard seed," he said, "ye shall say unto this mountain, Remove hence to yonder place; and it shall remove."[2]

The next step is to open our thought to what God knows and is causing man to be, even His own flawless image and likeness. We might ask in humility, "Father, what *is* going on?" Right back comes the answer to our prayer. Nothing is going on but God imparting good to His spiritual idea, man and the universe.

All real life inheres in God, Life. When understood to be all-powerful and omniactive, divine Life activates, regulates, harmonizes every organ and function of the human body. The textbook of Christian Science, *Science and Health* by Mary Baker Eddy, contains these statements: "Immortal Mind, governing all, must be acknowledged as supreme in the physical realm, so-called, as well as in the spiritual."[3] And, "Immortal Mind feeds the body with supernal freshness and fairness, supplying it with beautiful images of thought and destroying the woes of sense which each day brings to a nearer tomb."[4]

As we surrender frightened, agitated thoughts of disease to the serene, harmonious ideas coming to us from divine Truth, Life, and Love, the distress fades into nothingness, the disease loses its seeming reality, and the body assumes its normal state.

A student of Christian Science had an ugly growth on her leg. For four and a half years she had prayed about it in Christian Science; however, the growth remained just as ugly as ever. She often wondered why it didn't disappear, but since it didn't trouble her too much, she was rather apathetic over it.

Then one day as she sat praying over another situation, it became very clear to her that God alone is the cause of man's existence, and that unless God causes something, man cannot experience it. (Here was the self-assertive divine Principle making itself felt and known in individual consciousness.)

As she let this healing truth permeate her thinking, her eyes dropped to this ugly growth.

Truth was brilliant in her thought. It unfolded to her somewhat in this way: "Physical sense testimony says the growth is there, says I can see it and feel it, but my spiritual sense is saying it isn't there. What is true? If the very God of all the earth tells me it's not there, shouldn't I believe Him? And if He didn't put it there, how *can* it be there?"

There was no question left in the woman's mind. Because Principle is the only cause and is entirely good, the growth was not there.

Feeling released by this understanding, she suddenly knew what she'd been doing wrong all these years. She had been trying to use Truth to remove a physical condition, instead of surrendering her sense of an actual physical condition to Truth.

With this realization she turned on the liar — the erroneous, material consciousness called in Christian Science mortal mind — and addressed it in its impersonal status as a mere belief suddenly deprived of its believer. "I know what you've been doing," she declared. "You've been claiming the ability to substitute your false sense of physical body-with-a-growth for my God-constituted knowledge of my eternal spiritual perfection. Well, you'll never do it again!"

These false thoughts, she knew, had never really been her thoughts and had never been manifested in a discordant condition. From then on she met every challenge with the spiritual facts. Many times a day the growth would come to her attention, but each time she would meet the mental imposition with confidence and joy. Denouncing the suggestion of disease as impersonal evil, belonging to no one, she would restate the fact that she had a God-constituted, spiritual body as perfect now as it would ever be, functioning under divine law.

At the end of five weeks there was still no change. A demon suggestion came to her: "This isn't doing you any good." She laughed right out loud. "Oh, you're mistaken," she replied. "It's doing me a world of good. But if you keep coming for five hundred years, my answer will still be the same. You're not my thinking, and you can't describe my condition. I am as harmonious and safe as God."

That was the last time the growth ever came to her attention. The next time she was aware of this area of her body, the skin was clear and perfect. The growth had disappeared.

What if one's problem is a discordant relationship or a business problem? Would the basic approach be the same? It would. Surrender to the Principle of all true being, the one and only Mind, would necessitate a yielding up of belief in inharmony and conflict between individual personalities, as well as belief in many limited, finite minds.

Healing in Christian Science is a challenge, but one can approach every problem with a joyful sense of dominion and power. One actually has all the power of the universe behind his right efforts to do good, and a demonstration of divine might blesses everyone involved in the case, known or unknown to us.

The material view of man is entirely different from the view set forth in Genesis 1. Clearly a choice needs to be made between acceptance of this mistaken, discordant view and the spiritual idea of man as God-motivated, God-controlled, and God-blessed. Once one makes this choice, holds steadfastly to Principle, good, as the only cause, and lives accordingly, nothing can hinder his spiritual advancement and his demonstration of healing.

[1]See Gen. 1:26, 27, 31.   [2]Matt. 17:20.   [3]*Science and Health*, p. 427.   [4]*Ibid.*, p. 248.

Spiritual origin and childbirth

For prospective parents, the understanding of man's spiritual origin in God, Mind, can be an inspiring foundation for prayer.

The months prior to the birth of a child give parents the opportunity to understand more fully the fatherhood and motherhood of God and to see with clarity man's actual origin, substance, heritage, form, identity, individuality, and nature as spiritual. This understanding serves as a protection to the entire experience, lifting it above the possibility of chance to the natural manifestation of divine law. Seeing that man is truly born "not of blood, nor of the will of the flesh, nor of the will of man, but of God"[1] helps overrule supposed physiological laws, with their sometimes detrimental effects, and opens thought to seeing birth not as a material process but as the reflection of the creative power of divine Spirit.

Building on the understanding that man's origin is in Spirit, we come to see that man's substance is not subject to discord or malfunction. It expresses the freshness, beauty, purity, and immortality of Spirit. Christ Jesus brought this truth to light through his healing works.

Understanding that man's preexistence and eternal continuance are in Spirit displaces the false sense of identity as formed materially and therefore subject to chance or unpredictability. To see the substance of a child's being as timeless, as eternal, as infinite, is to free him from apparent material laws regarding substance. As Mary Baker Eddy states in *Science and Health,* "Spirit and its formations are the only realities of being."[2]

The true identity of a child is nourished by everlasting Father-Mother Love, is established by unerring, fixed Principle, and expresses the perfection of endless Life. His identity is inseparable from God. It evidences the nature and action of the one Mind. Man is the individual expression of God. Goodness, joy, intelligence, beauty, wisdom, activity — all the creator's qualities — identify him. Each individuality is loved, cherished, and indispensable to the Father's allness. There can be no unwanted child in the expression of God's fullness.

As the birth commences, parents can rely on the fact that true creation is spiritual, governed harmoniously by divine Principle. In the consciousness of divine Love's presence, there is no fear of an opposing force or law to obstruct the birth. Since God's law alone is supreme, no other supposed law has actual power to interfere with the birth process.

Spiritual preparation through prayer has been a natural and essential part of our family's development. This has particularly been true in the times before the births of my children and has helped to free me from fear and discomfort. The births of the first two children were quick and free of pain. However, with the third child, the birth started forward briefly, and then for almost a day nothing significant happened. The Christian Science practitioner who was helping me through prayer quoted this statement from *Science and Health:* "The power of Christian Science and divine Love is omnipotent. It is indeed adequate to unclasp the hold and to destroy disease, sin, and death."[3] As I hung up the telephone, I asked in prayerful thought, "What is holding up this birth?" The answer that came was that no material law had any hold on God's child and that His child was governed by the law and activity of Spirit. Within a minute of that firm declaration of truth, the birth proceeded.

We were having the child at home and had the help of a Christian Science nurse. And we engaged a doctor to be present at the birth. Within an hour or so our child arrived, but the doctor wasn't able to be there, although he did come within thirty minutes. The Christian Science nurse was present and gently took care of the child. The truth that the practitioner had shared from *Science and Health* was just exactly what was needed to bring harmony to the birth, and that truth continued to light the way as the situation developed.

A medical nurse who worked with the doctor came to our home in the morning to do a routine check of the baby. She found that its heart-rate pattern was questionable. The doctor insisted that we bring the baby into his office immediately for a further check. When we agreed, we were informed that the child could very well have a serious heart defect. We were strongly urged to have a specialist test the child, and the doctor reiterated the consequences of not doing this.

To parents of a new child, this verdict could have been devastating, coming on the heels of so much joy and gratitude for the birth itself. But all those nine months, and even months before that, had been spent in opening thought to God's creation and beholding the truth of His offspring. It had been a cherished, consecrated time of prayer. I was fortified with the spiritual understanding that I had gained during that time and felt confident that the child's life was governed by divine law. I had come to see that the very source of the child's being was Spirit and that the child therefore had only the perfect substance of Spirit, expressing the perfect action of Spirit. I realized that the integrity of what was called heart action had a divine source; it wasn't in matter. I saw too that this action was preserved through the divine law of Life.

Humbly listening for God's wisdom in the situation, we took the baby to have the tests. After the examination, the specialist pronounced the child perfectly healthy. Needless to say, we rejoiced with much gratitude!

An understanding of man's spiritual origin brought to bear on childbirth brings great blessings, because it lifts off material theories and reveals man as perfect, governed by the law of Spirit.

[1]John 1:13. [2]*Science and Health,* p. 264. [3]*Ibid.,* p. 412.

What does it mean to be a real woman?

"Now there's a *real* woman!" How often have you heard that said about some attractive woman? But is that true? Is our womanhood (or manhood for that matter) dependent upon our physical appearance and attractiveness to the opposite sex? Many television programs, movies, books, and advertising campaigns try to tell us "yes." However, more and more people are experiencing the unhappy effects of such an outlook. Feelings of loneliness, lust, emptiness, helplessness, and obsession with the body often drive them to seek a deeper view of who they really are. I know!

As I entered adulthood, I brought with me the misconception that sensuality was part of true womanhood. The more adult and "womanly" I viewed myself, the easier it became to relax my moral standard until chastity was a thing of the past, even though

I knew that it wasn't in accord with what I'd learned in Christian Science. Throughout my single years, I had the desire deep down to be lifted above this immoral activity. I often struggled alternately with self-justification and then guilt. I knew that I really needed to base my moral standard on an understanding of God and of spiritual law, rather than on human will or opinion (which I found collapsed during times of temptation).

I continued my attendance and membership in my local Christian Science branch church, although I was not active. (I will always be grateful for that anchor of branch church membership, which helped keep me from drifting too far.) I knew that if I allowed the guilt and self-condemnation I felt to separate me from the one thing that would help save me, I might never gain my dominion.

I eventually met and married my husband and felt that the problem was solved. I now had the protection and commitment of marriage to sanction our sexual relations. But sensuality still seemed very important to my sense of womanhood.

The first few years of our marriage were filled with discord and dissatisfaction. Then, over a period of about one year, I found myself strongly attracted to two men with whom I worked. I became involved in relationships that came near to breaking the Seventh Commandment, "Thou shalt not commit adultery."[1] At times the physical attraction seemed overwhelming. But an overriding love for God, love of my husband, and the desire to do what I knew was morally right enabled me to break off the first relationship. When I found myself again strongly tempted, I knew I had to go deeper than outward obedience to the law of God, as important as that is. I had to confront this notion that physical appearance and attraction were what made me a true woman.

It was my husband's quiet example that gradually led me to a higher understanding of man's spiritual identity and that broke the hypnotic pull of sensuality. I had made him aware of these struggles and asked him to help me through them. Because he is a student of Christian Science, I hoped that he would be able to see this challenge as a deeper issue than just a frustrated, unfaithful wife. His amazing grace during this difficult time revealed to me what a real man is. The qualities of integrity, patience, moral strength, and uncondemning love that he lived far outshone the good looks that had seemed so attractive. I began to recognize the real spiritual nature of man and to value this expression of true manhood.

As I gained greater conviction and spiritual understanding, the second relationship was also ended harmoniously, although I continued working with both men. As I continued to pray and grow in my understanding of my true identity, I thought a lot about the answer to a question "What is man?" found in *Science and Health*. It seemed especially helpful in this particular case to think of the word *woman* whenever *man* was mentioned, since Mrs. Eddy uses "man" generically. I saw more clearly than ever before that woman "is idea, the image, of Love; [she] is not physique. [She] is the compound idea of God, including all right ideas . . . ."[2] Each person's real individuality stems solely from God, Soul, Spirit. Because God is Spirit, our real identity must be wholly spiritual, the reflection of God's nature. This nature is pure and good and innocent. Such qualities as beauty, grace, love, and intuition, usually associated with womanhood, have nothing to do with a material body. Rightly seen, they are wholly the manifestation of Soul, Spirit.

I also saw that as God's expression I could include only "right ideas." Sensual, selfish beliefs are not from God; therefore I didn't need to hold on to them and they could not hold on to me. In the *Manual of The Mother Church,* Mrs. Eddy calls on each member of her Church "to defend himself daily against aggressive mental suggestion...."[3] And that's really all physical attraction is, aggressive *mental* suggestion. There is no powerful physical chemistry between material human bodies. The seeming attraction begins and ends in *thought.* And it is in thought that we must combat any temptation to break any of God's commandments.

We may be tempted to blame God for our sensuality. Maybe we've heard or said, "I can't help myself! God made me this way!" Would God, who is Love, knowingly create man so that he couldn't help sinning and then punish him for committing the sin? The Bible sets us straight on this point when it explains, "Let no man say when he is tempted, I am tempted of God: for God cannot be tempted with evil, neither tempteth he any man: but every man is tempted, when he is drawn away of his own lust, and enticed."[4]

Another aggressive mental suggestion I uncovered in my thinking was the concept that we are animals, the "human animal" as people often refer to humankind. Well, the man of God's creating is *not* an animal! He is not made up of animal urges and reactions. This belief is exactly the opposite of the true view of man as God's pure, sinless image and likeness, the spiritual view described in the first chapter of Genesis. And in the New Testament, the Bible warns us of the consequences of thinking of ourselves in carnal, animal terms: "For to be carnally minded is death; but to be spiritually minded is life and peace."[5] Our real, spiritual nature as the pure creation and reflection of God is tangibly manifested in us as we claim this fact ourselves and reflect it in our thoughts and actions. We can know and prove that we are impelled only by divine Love, not animal lust. The presence of divine Love in our thought fills the emptiness of sensuality with a warm, lasting peace and tender affection founded on purity and goodness.

At times it may seem to be a struggle to rise above the magnetism of the so-called animal nature. But, as we grasp the truth of our real spiritual identity and strive to demonstrate it in our lives, that magnetic pull ceases to dominate — and appetites and passions are brought under Christly discipline and control. To win this battle we need to be alert to the continual barrage of mental suggestions that would have us believe we are animals, controlled by physicality. We need to be more selective in the television, movies, and books we use for entertainment and the advertising campaigns we respond to. Do they reflect the higher nature of men and women, or are they glorifying and appealing to a lower, animal nature? Do they stir spiritual inspiration or physical sensation? This isn't being stuffy or prudish. It's refusing to be sold the empty bill of goods that says men, women, and even children are sensuous humans governed by animal urges.

It has been about six years since this experience occurred. Since then my marriage has blossomed into the sweetest, most satisfying relationship I could have imagined. What a joy to be able to recognize a "real man" when I see one! How grateful I am to know finally what it means to be a "real woman."

[1]Ex. 20:14. [2]*Science and Health*, p. 475. [3]*Manual*, Art. VIII, Sect. 6. [4]James 1:13, 14. [5]Rom. 8:6.

Women's rights and true womanhood

Increasingly, today's women, and many men, too, are confidently claiming the undeniable right of women to be accepted as equal with men. The intelligence, business sense, artistic talent, and spiritual insight of women, as well as their right to follow a career with opportunities for advancement equal to those of their male colleagues, are being more widely recognized and acknowledged. Perhaps this reflects a growing conviction in society that women have a vital part to play in our world in *all* walks of life.

When we look at this issue from a spiritual perspective, the essential nature of true womanhood stands out, generous and compassionate, patient and perceptive. The qualities of true womanhood — and manhood — are really inherent in all of us, because our genuine selfhood is the reflection of our Father-Mother God. Understanding and claiming this spiritual fact can enlarge the horizon of our thinking with a powerfully freeing effect on our lives.

The spiritual perspective on womanhood can be found in the Bible. For example, the first chapter of Genesis describes the nature of man in these words: "So God created man in his own image, in the image of God created he him; male and female created he them."[1] The New Testament tells us God is Spirit; thus this verse can be seen as bringing out the spiritual nature of man, the indestructible individuality of each one of us.

We may be used to thinking of God as Father, and Christ Jesus referred to "my Father," "your Father," and "our Father." But the Bible points out the cherishing and nurturing qualities of God as divine Love, as well as the protecting and guiding qualities — the motherly as well as the fatherly attributes of our Father-Mother God. For instance, in Deuteronomy, Moses vividly portrays the deliverer of the children of Israel as like a mother eagle, carrying her young to safety on her wings; and the author in Isaiah reassures his troubled hearers that their Lord will comfort them as a mother. And Jesus certainly lived the compassion and tender care that he taught.

Each of us, then, as the image of God, must inevitably include the feminine as well as the masculine qualities of the heavenly Parent in complete spiritual individuality. Realizing this spiritual fact enables us to live more of this real selfhood in daily life, to discover within ourselves a natural capacity for both authority and tenderness, compassion and strength.

Accepting the purely spiritual nature of their real being encourages women to claim exemption from the suffering that is often thought to be natural at different times in women's lives. This happened in my own experience. I found myself for no apparent reason acutely unhappy, struggling with depression and loneliness. My sense of isolation was such that I did not feel able even to confide in my husband, who was aware of my distress and more than ready to give me his loving support. I prayed earnestly to understand more of the ever-presence of a wholly good and loving God who cared for me and would not permit anything that could cause me suffering or take away my joy and peace of mind. One day in despair I simply cried out to God for help.

Shortly afterward it suddenly became clear to me that this was a symptom of menopause, and I set about finding the specific spiritual antidote for this difficulty.

I turned to the familiar verse from Genesis already quoted. This reassured me that, as the image of God, I reflect the masculine and feminine qualities of God in perfect balance, a settled state that could not be disturbed; that because my true selfhood is spiritual, I do not have to conform to material, so-called laws that prescribe suffering at different stages of physical maturity. I recognized that this is true for all women and that I could claim the right to freedom for myself and for womankind.

Almost immediately the depression lifted, and I felt comforted and more cheerful. Also, I was able to discuss the situation naturally with my husband and receive his support. However, this was not the end of the story.

I had recently completed a three-year term as a Reader in my branch Church of Christ, Scientist. I was looking forward to having even more time for study of the Bible and the writings of Mary Baker Eddy, which that work had involved. It had been a satisfying and very busy three years, spent caring for my family and also from time to time looking after other relatives, in addition to my church commitment. By the end of my term, our children had left home for college and careers, and I was not needed nearly so much by other family members. Our home and church work kept me occupied, but I felt underemployed simply looking after my husband and myself. The study I had been looking forward to so eagerly suddenly seemed pointless. I was not contributing financially to our home, and I seemed to have no useful part to play in the family, or indeed anywhere. An empty future stretched ahead of me.

Holding on to the recently awakened sense of my complete spiritual identity, however, I soon realized that this picture was actually just another restricted view of womanhood, portraying a woman's interests as confined to a single role or a particular routine.

I realized that I was free to accept or to challenge this concept. It was clear that I needed to learn more about the true status of woman in the light of spiritual creation. I went back to the Bible and to Mrs. Eddy's writings to understand more of woman, the feminine nature, gender, and so on, but for some time I felt uninspired, and the thought of uselessness persisted.

Then one day, in the course of my reading I came across Mrs. Eddy's use of the phrases "the womanhood of God" (*Christian Healing*) and "the manhood and womanhood of God" (*The First Church of Christ, Scientist, and Miscellany*). I suddenly saw clearly that the nature of God not only *combines* masculine and feminine elements but that they are *all* valuable and important. The qualities of intuition, gentleness, and grace, of intelligence, strength, and courage, are *all* essential for the complete reflection of the character of God, the fullness of Spirit.

Traditionally, in many cultures the role of men as providers and protectors has been dominant, with women taking a subordinate position. With this in mind, I looked at the story of Adam and Eve in the second chapter of Genesis. Here Adam is reported to be created by "the Lord God" (not the God of the first account of creation) as a material being. The woman is later created, almost as an afterthought, in order to fill a need of Adam for a help and companion. In the following chapter, the ancient writer makes plain the woman's subordinate role, her total dependence on her husband, and her very limited prospects. It is as if the woman were firmly put in her place and expected to stay there.

However, the subservience of an Eve bears no resemblance whatever to the spiritual status of man — male and female — in the spiritual creation described in the first chapter of Genesis. We have no legitimate grounds for devaluing femininity and denying the womanhood of God.

Reasoning along these lines, I felt a new, tremendous freedom. I walked around the house, joyfully repeating to myself that God did not make man first and woman second. I did not have to accept a fictional Eve-like role. I had native worth as a daughter of God, and I had my place in God's scheme of things. This was not simply wishful thinking or morale boosting but a spiritual *fact*. My value as an individual was not diminished because my family needed less of my time.

Mrs. Eddy believed firmly in the importance of the family and a woman's contribution to its stability as wife and mother. Yet she did not envisage women's restriction to that sphere. In a pamphlet called *No and Yes* she wrote, "In natural law and in religion the right of woman to fill the highest measure of enlightened understanding and the highest places in government, is inalienable, and these rights are ably vindicated by the noblest of both sexes."[2] True manhood and womanhood complement and support one another; they do not compete, nor conflict, nor elbow one another aside.

One dictionary definition of the word *career* is "course, or progress through life." Trying to live the completeness of the character of God, expressing our own unique blend of divine qualities, masculine and feminine, so as to be an influence for peace and stability, is a challenging course through life. At the same time, it must surely be the most worthwhile full-time employment we can have, irrespective of our occupation, trade, vocation.

In my own case, while I felt considerably strengthened by this new evaluation of myself, the suggestion of uselessness returned in one form or another for some time and had to be continually refuted in the light of my newfound spiritual understanding and through persistent study. At the same time, there was a steady improvement in my experience. Of course, I found that I still had a part to play in supporting our children and enjoying their friendship. I recognized that working for my church was not a second-rate substitute for a "proper job" but an important contribution toward healing problems in our community. I stopped feeling that I was inferior because I was not earning a salary. I took up other interests. Most of all, I relished the time spent praying and studying and saw it as an opportunity to expand my concept of motherhood, to include the community and the world in my prayers.

A few months later I discovered that I had become entitled to a modest pension because of the years I had been employed before my marriage. I received a sum for the accumulated benefit, and a regular payment continues. This was as unexpected as it was welcome, and it enables me to contribute financially to our home.

True womanhood is one of our natural, vast resources of wealth — spiritually, morally, and practically. Whether we're women or men, no matter what our current occupation, we each have a unique contribution to make to the welfare of the universal family.

[1]Gen. 1:27. [2]*No and Yes,* p. 45.

"The 'male and female' of God's creating"

Several cases of sexual harassment in the workplace were covered recently by the media, triggering discussions of woman's position in society. Numerous injustices were uncovered, such as less pay for the same work, and violence against women. Even before this discussion in the media, when I had had to deal with such discrimination quite a bit myself, I had come to the conclusion that confrontation between the sexes cannot solve these problems.

Some time later, my husband introduced me to Christian Science and its textbook, *Science and Health with Key to the Scriptures* by Mary Baker Eddy. In that book I found the spiritual interpretation of the Lord's Prayer, the first line of which seemed especially remarkable and revolutionary to me at the time. It reads, "Our Father which art in heaven, *Our Father-Mother God, all-harmonious.*"[1]

Here, God was portrayed as both Father and Mother, masculine and feminine! I found this thought fascinating and marvelous.

The Bible records, in Genesis, "God created man in his own image, in the image of God he him; male and female created he them."[2] In the Christian Science textbook Mrs. Eddy writes as follows about this Bible passage: "To emphasize this momentous thought, it is repeated that God made man in His own image, to reflect the divine Spirit. It follows that *man* is a generic term. Masculine, feminine, and neuter genders are human concepts."[3]

So if we are to recognize our spiritual completeness as the male and female of God's creating, we must lay aside all mortal notions of the division of qualities according to gender.

God, Spirit, is described in the Bible as love, soul, truth, life, lawgiver, as the Almighty. He is all-knowing and supreme, replete with qualities such as mercy, goodness, justice, strength, tenderness, gentleness, and patience. The Bible also says that God is the only creator of man and that His creation is perfect and good. It follows from this that man cannot possess anything that does not come from God.

In contrast to this, in the second and third chapters of Genesis we read of a material act of creation and the fall of man. This account ends with Adam and Eve being banished from paradise and condemned—in a gender-specific way, so to speak.[4] The Bible tells us that God cursed them in this way: "Unto the woman he said, I will greatly multiply thy sorrow and thy conception; in sorrow thou shalt bring forth children; and thy desire shall be to thy husband, and he shall rule over thee." Nor did Adam fare any better. He was condemned to a life of sorrow and labor before dying and returning to dust.

Aren't these images familiar? A woman sacrificing herself in sorrow for her children and dependent on her husband, and a man working to feed his family by the sweat of his brow. This was supposed to be a punishment for both!

We can regard these images as figments of mortal, limited thinking that have nothing in common with divine reality. They are the result of thought that is separated from God. As God's perfect, spiritual likeness, man does not have biological attributes; rather, he reflects divine qualities, which we characterize as being masculine and feminine in nature. Each of us can lay claim to all these qualities and can express them fully. In other words, there is no such thing as a woman without initiative or intelligence, nor is there any such thing as a man who is uncompassionate, uncaring.

Our Master, Christ Jesus, expressed both masculine and feminine qualities in perfect harmony. The Bible reports his great gentleness and compassion as well as his clarity and courage. He accepted only God's perfect likeness, not allowing prejudice or preconceived notions to enter into his appraisal of others. His caring extended equally to men and women.

By rejecting limiting clichéd roles in our prayers and replacing them with the divine truth about the completeness of man, we help those suffering under such prejudices. We can also experience healing for ourselves.

I found this out myself when a previously diagnosed uterine cyst started to cause me pain again, and I became increasingly fearful. In the time since the diagnosis I had learned of Christian Science, and I decided to heal the condition through prayer. I acknowledged that I was created perfect and that no malfunctioning could creep into the action of the divine law. I also prayed to understand better that I could not be susceptible to certain diseases because of my gender, as is frequently asserted in press reports. As a complete idea of

God, I incorporated only good masculine and feminine qualities. The pain stopped very quickly after that, and I felt the fear had been overcome as well.

The next day, however, a friend of mine telephoned. She had a similar problem and was going to have a small operation for it. No sooner had I hung up than massive fear overwhelmed me. Immediately, I turned to God in prayer with all my heart. Prompted by a testimony about the healing of a disease common to women, which I had read in a previous issue of this magazine, I studied, among other things, this passage from Revelation: "And there appeared a great wonder in heaven; a woman clothed with the sun, and the moon under her feet, and upon her head a crown of twelve stars."[5]

The moon is widely known as a symbol for femininity. It is said to have a bearing on the menstrual cycle and to have other disruptive effects on sensitive people. But since the woman is "clothed with the sun" — divine light, Life, Truth, and Love — and has the "moon under her feet," that meant to me that she has dominion over all the claims that are generally attributed to her sex. It isn't the moon — the material claim — that illuminates her and makes up the nature of her being, but divine Truth. She reflects only this divine light. From this, I saw that all women — including me and my friend really were made to express God. This realization completely dispelled my fear for myself and my friend. When she called again four days later, I was happy to learn that she had recovered quickly and was able to go home earlier than expected.

Of course, the way I chose to deal with this physical problem was totally different from my friend's, because Christian Science does not combine prayer and medicine. By relying solely on prayer I was healed and so proved in my own way the truth of this statement in *Science and Health:* "Let us accept Science, relinquish all theories based on sense-testimony, give up imperfect models and illusive ideals; and so let us have one God, one Mind, and that one perfect, producing His own models of excellence. Let the 'male and female' of God's creating appear."[6]

My experience proves that we are not helplessly at the mercy of "imperfect models." Fully claiming God's qualities brings infinite blessings to us and to others.

[1]*Science and Health*, p. 16. [2]Gen. 1:27. [3]*Science and Health*, p. 516. [4]See Gen. 3:16–19. [5]Rev. 12:1. [6]*Science and Health*, p. 249.

AFTERWORD

Ideas expressed in this publication are based on the teachings of Christian Science, founded on the life and works of Christ Jesus.

Christian Science is fully explained in Mary Baker Eddy's book, *Science and Health with Key to the Scriptures*, which may be purchased from any Christian Science Reading Room. Open to the public, Reading Rooms can usually be located through the local telephone directory.

PS9512020